Yan d'Albert

ARGAN OIL

The healing gold
of the desert

Yan d'Albert

ARGAN OIL

The healing gold
of the desert

series biosol

edition
SOL

The informations and recommendations presented here are proofed with the best knowledge and belief, nevertheless the author and publisher does not take any liability for any damages which may be suffered as a direct or indirect result of the here presented applications. In any case observe the limits of self-treatment and with symptoms of illness make use of professional diagnosis and therapy by medical or natural help.

English edition: ARGAN OIL – The healing gold of the desert. German original edition: ARGAN ÖL – Die wunderbare Heilkraft des Wüstengoldes. English reader: Caroline Neumüller, info@caroline-neumueller.de. © edition SOL Yan d'Albert, Bergisch Gladbach 2014/2016. All rights reserved. www.editionsol.de, www.yandalbert.de

ISBN-13: 978-1523614875
ISBN-10: 1523614870

BismiLlâh ir-Rahmân ir-Rahîem

In the name of Allâh, the Most Gracious, the Most Merciful

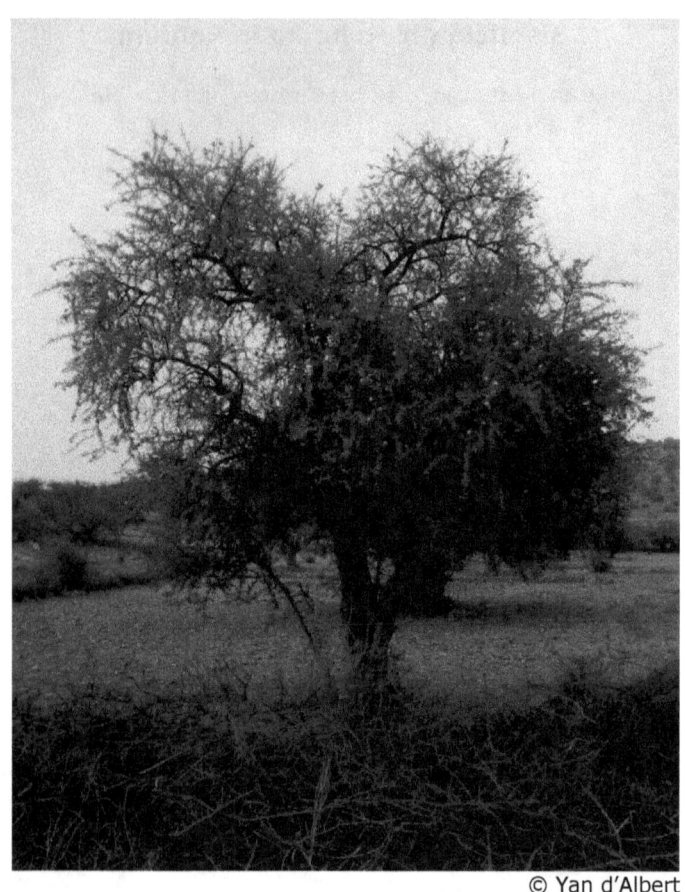

© Yan d'Albert

Argan tree near Tiout (South Morocco)

INDEX

MY WAY TO ARGAN ... **8**
THE PLANT **10**
OCCURENCES **12**
THE PRODUCTION **14**
COMPOSITION AND MEDICAL EFFECTS **16**
PREVENTION OF ILLNESSES **17**
REGISTER OF APPLICATIONS **18**
COSMETICS **20**
CUISINE **23**
RECIPE **24**
DISTRIBUTION **25**

MY WAY TO ARGAN ...

Once in the South Moroccan holiday resort *Agadir* I met my dear wife Hajiba. She stems from a Berber family, which carries on the trade of extraction of Argan. Naturally I came into contact with Argan.

It was the first time when I travelled by taxi to the native town of my wife. I looked out of the window and couldn't believe my eyes: Everywhere in the trees goats sat plucking leaves and fruits. "Argan, Argan!" the taxi driver called out and pointed with the finger at the trees. So these are said to be Argan trees, about whose oil my wife raved about. Soon the golden yellow oil fascinated me, too. Never before I became acquainted with such a fine extremely versatile oil. Whether in the cuisine as a salad oil, for skin and hair as a care product or internally applied, I was deeply impressed by the taste and wonderful effects of Argan, I had the privilege to experience it more and more.

With reference to medicine, cosmetics and nutrition Argan oil is one of the most precious and most effective oils of the world. This "liquid gold of the desert" is a universal miracle against various troubles and illnesses. Through internal and external application it works preventatively and keeps the body fit. Today one recognizes these beneficial effects more and more, also in the west.

Argan - what a marvellous plant, what a benefit for mankind! With this publication I have tried to summarize the most important and essential facts about this miracle oil.

My writing may serve as an impulse for pleasure, well-being and cure by Argan oil. A lot of people may become and remain healthy by its power, as God wills.

8

And the same I wish to you

with all my heart

Yours

Yan d'Albert

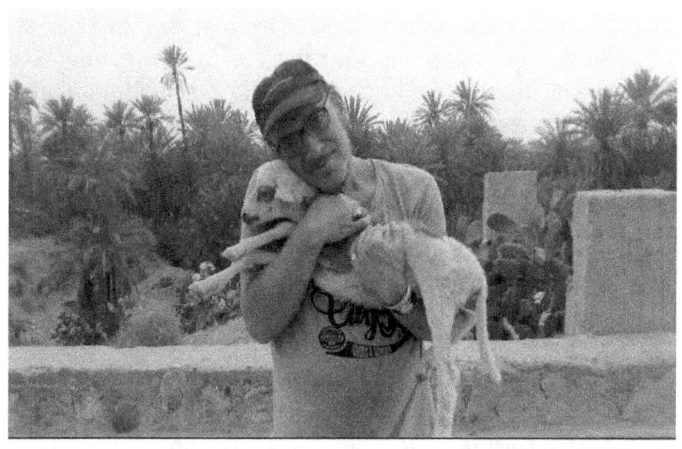

A little lamb from Tiout - so cute!

THE PLANT

The Argan oil tree, whose scientific Latin name is *Argania spinosa,* belongs to the oldest trees in the world. For over 80 million years they have grown in Morocco's Southwest, in the area of *Essaouira, Agadir* and *Taroudant*, at the *High Atlas*.

The Argan tree reaches a height of up to 10 m, a girth of up to 15 m and can become between 200 and 400 years old. It requires very little water and survives also temperatures up to over 50 degrees Celsius. It has the ability to bear fruits several times a year. The olive-like fruits are not edible for humans. The goats however are crazy about them as well as the leaves. From the fruits the precious Argan oil is won. The pressing residues from the oil extraction are traditionally used as animal food and also as remedies for animal wounds. The wood of the Argan trees serve as fuel as well.

A long time ago Moroccos natives, the *Amazighs,* began to use the precious oil as elixir of life. Until today it is part of the tradition of the Berbers to give the bride Argan oil on her wedding. The family of the bride brings the nuts; then the villagers produce the oil.

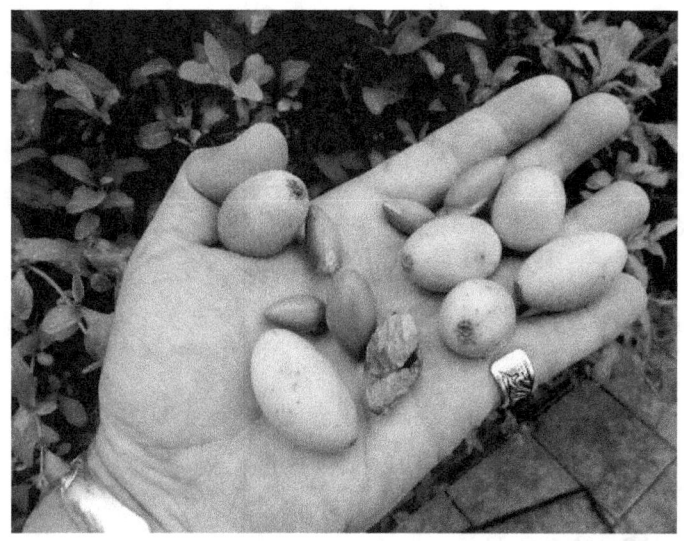

Yellow Argan fruits and their brown nuts

OCCURRENCES

The dear God verily means it well with the South Moroccan Berbers, because Argan trees grow actually *only* in the area of the Southern Atlas Mountains. Argan plays an important role with the people in its origin region. Especially the oil extraction is an important source of revenue for the structurally weak areas. 80 percent are accounted for manual work. The Moroccans tried to plant Argan trees also in other areas of Morocco, however without success. Since 1998 the biosphere reserve of the Argan trees is under the protection of the *Unesco*. For example Germany promotes projects to the afforestation and supports foundations like "LA FONDATION POUR L'ARGANIER."

The Argan tree is an ecologically important component of the dry ecosystem in Morocco's Southwest. The planting of Argan trees counteracts the soil erosion and desertification. So some initiatives and cooperatives strive to protect and to use tree plantings to plant new ones.

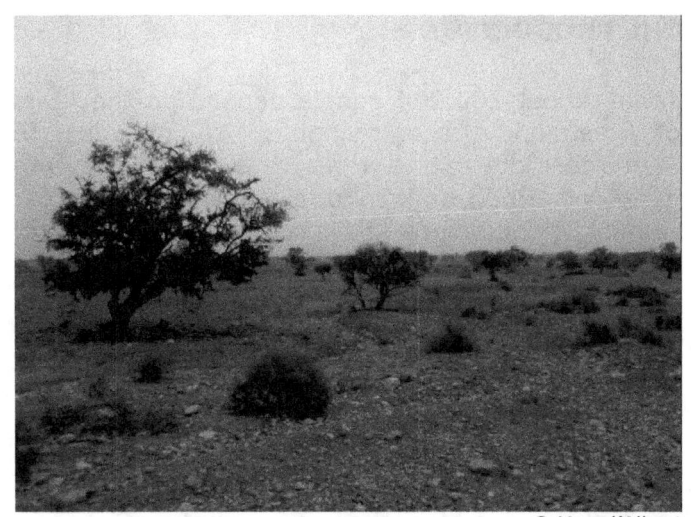

Argan trees, as far as the eye can see …

THE PRODUCTION

Today about 200.000 people depend on the fruits of Argan and the extraction of it. From July to September the nuts are harvested. Then they are dried and stored. In laborious handicraft the Berber women manufacture the precious oil. The hard nuts are opened between two stones. Afterwards they are lightly roasted, mixed with water and finally processed with a stone mill to a semolina-like slurry. Finally, the women press the oil from it by hand. For the extraction of one liter Argan oil a woman requires 50 kg of the fruit and she needs nearly a whole day for this work. Most of the Berber women involved at the not-industrial production joined together as cooperatives.

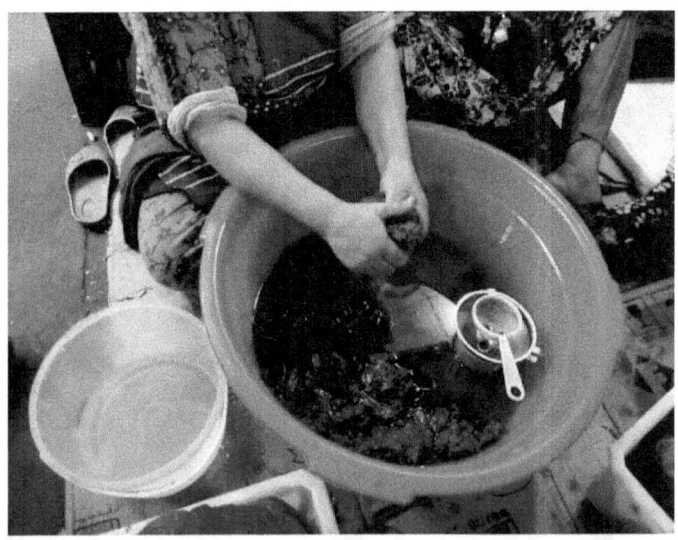

© Yan d'Albert

Argan oil extraction is only possible through manual labour and is made by Berber women with much effort and love.

14

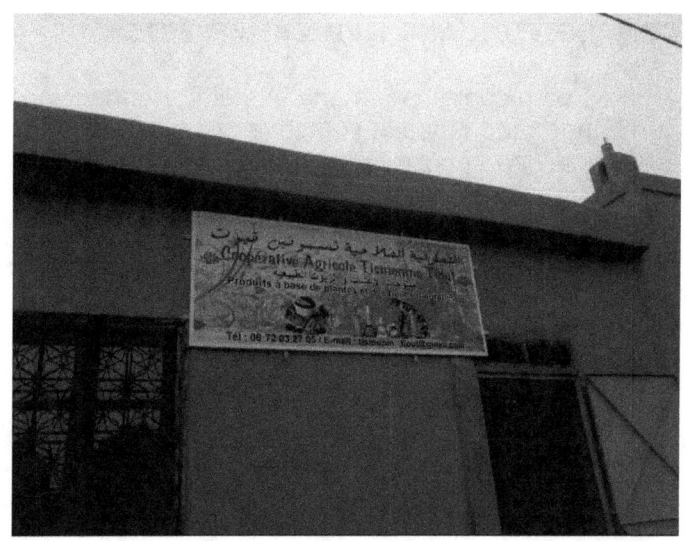

The Argan cooperative in Tiout: "Cooperative Agricole Tismonine Tioute"

COMPOSITION AND MEDICAL EFFECTS

Argan oil contains many health enhancing, nurturing and healing active substances. It possesses an enormous nutritional-physiological valency and a high concentration, namely 80 percent of healthy unsaturated fatty acids (radical quenchers).

It is rich in **tocopherols** and therefore it contains a high Vitamin E content. This means that these anti-oxidants can intercept aggressive oxygen molecules in the body and help strengthen our immune system.

Further in the Argan oil are **phytosterols** (schottenols and spinasterols), which, scientifically proven, have an anti-tumor activity, finally prevent the growth of cancer cells.

Further components in the oil are **querzetins** and **myriezetins** which are effective against bacteria and fungi. There are also **triterpenalcohols** in it, which protect the skin and have a disinfectant, anti-inflammatory and wound healing effect.

PREVENTION OF ILLNESSES

It is scientifically proven that there is a five times lower cancer risk through the taking of Argan oil. Already the internal application of one teaspoon of pure Argan oil three times a day lowers the risk to catch various illnesses up to cancer.

REGISTER OF APPLICATIONS

Doctors and immunologists attest, that no other oil supplies our immune system with such valuable substances like Argan oil, with regular food intake or through cosmetic treatment.

The most important applications in keywords are listed in the following register:

Acne
Allergy
Alzheimer
Anti-Aging
Arteriosclerosis
Birth problems
Cancer (reduction of the cancer risk)
Cellulite
Chickenpox
Cholesterol levels (elevated)
Dementia
Digestion
Eczemas
Fertility
Hair care
Hair (dry or brittle)
Hair loss
Heart and circulatory problems
Heart attack
Hemorrhoids
Immune system (strengthening)
Itching
Joint illnesses, joint pains
Metabolic disorder

Menopause
Nails (brittle)
Neurodermatitis
Parkinson
Pimple scars
Pregnancy (better childbirth by usage of Argan oil)
Psoriasis
Rheumatism and rheumatic diseases
Skin ageing
Skin protection against sun
Skin (dry, broken or raw)
Stretch marks
Stress
Sunburn
Sun protection
Well-being (in general)
Wrinkles
Wounds (desinfection and cure)

COSMETICS

SKIN CARE OIL - ANTI-AGING

Why do the Berber women have such a young, wrinkle-free skin up until old age, despite hard work and permanently high solar radiation? The magical cure is: ARGAN OIL! The high content of unsaturated fatty acids and vitamin E supports the natural own protection of the skin and minimizes the risk of skin damages. Already one or two applications with a few drops a day are enough for the care and protection of the skin. As suntan oil it protects and tans.

HAIR CARE

Hair treatment

Argan oil is ideal for the universal hair care, because it contains valuable ingredients and a high vitamin E content. With Argan oil the hair preserves its moisture and protects from the formation of split ends. It boosts silkiness and natural sheen for dry and stressed hair.

Heat up the oil in a small bowl. Then you divide your hair with your fingers into medium thick strands and apply the Argan into the dry hair. After you comb your hair over your head with a comb or a brush and pack it in a warm towel. Allow to take effect for half an hour and finally wash the hair with a mild shampoo.

Hair massage

Argan oil is also well applicable for a scalp treatment, particularly useful for hair loss. Massage the heated up Argan oil softly into the scalp. Allow to take effect a half to one hour and at the end wash it with a mild shampoo.

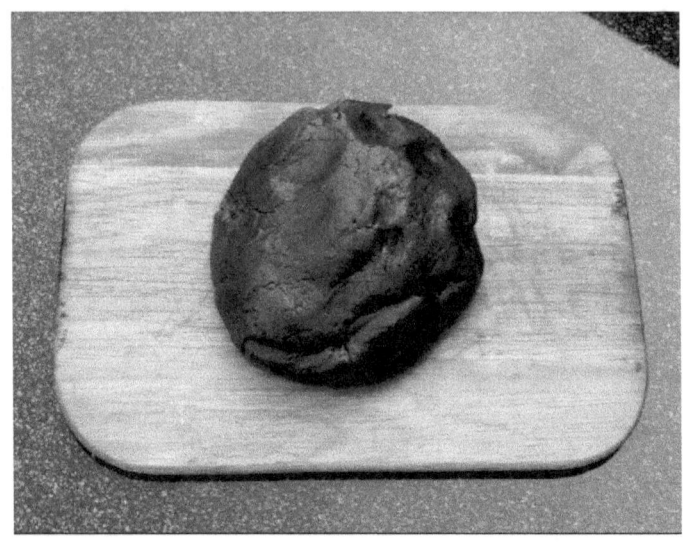

"Taksmout", the Argan nut paste, mixed with water, suitable also as face mask

CUISINE

Argan oil has developed into the sought-after gourmet edible oil. International star cooks
are very enthusiastic by the delicacy of Argan oil and it has become an irreplaceable component of their cuisines. Its fine nutty note, its pleasantly soft and oily flavor is ideally suited for cooking and seasoning, as oil for salads, soups, vegetables, fish, meat but also for sweet deserts.

Finally there is a traditional Berber recipe, with which a delicious dessert can be created with the use of Argan oil:

RECIPE

Amlou

Amlou is a delicious mixture of almonds, honey and Argan oil, which is suitable as bread spread or to grill dishes and Tajines. Amlou is known for its health promoting and aphrodisiacal effect.

Ingredients:

For about 400 g Amlou mixture
250 g whole almonds
1 tbs vegetable oil
100 ml Argan oil
4 tbs liquid honey
Salt

Give the almonds in a pot with boiling water. Blanch them, fill them into a sieve, drain them and let them cool down. Then peel them. Roast the almonds lightly at medium heat and let them cool down. Afterwards you give the almonds with the Argan oil and salt into a mixer and stir everything to a creamy mixture. Add the honey and mix it well. Finally you fill the mixture into a glass and store it in a cool place. Amlou keeps in the fridge for two months. If it should last longer, you leave out the honey in the preparation and add it shortly before consumption and mix it into the mixture. Serve Amlou with a real mint tea.

DISTRIBUTION

When buying Argan oil, you should make sure that it is 100 percent argan quality (without chemical additions or mixtures).

ARGAN SOL is known as the best Argan oil ever and is distributed as the **only** 100% organic (Bio)-Argan oil from lightly or not roasted Argan nuts, directly from the source, without further additions, handmade from Berber women in South Morocco with much effort and love.

Supply source:

ARGAN SOL
Yan d'Albert
Odenthaler St. 190
D-51467 Bergisch Gladbach
Phone: +49 2202 1085727
Mobile: +49 177 56 21773
www.editionsol.de
www.yandalbert.de
editionsol@t-online.de
yandalbert@t-online.de